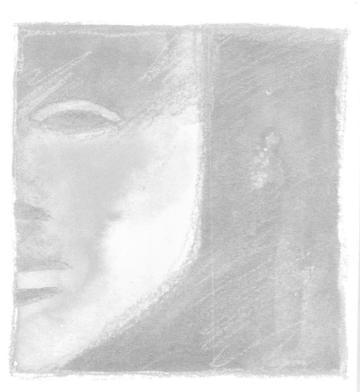

The Dougy Center for
Grieving Children,
3909 S.E. 52nd Ave.,
P.O. Box 86852,
Portland, OR 97286.

Phone:
503•775•5683

Written and printed in
the United States of
America.

ISBN 1-890534-00-5

Helping Children Cope with Death

Contents

This guidebook has been developed by **The Dougy Center,** *The National Center for Grieving Children & Families.* Since 1983, The Center has worked with thousands of children, teens and their adult family members who have experienced the death of a parent, adult caregiver, sibling or teen friend.

The information presented here is compiled from the real-life stories of the children, teens and their parents. Too often our society fails to support young people and adults after a death. They experience isolation and misunderstanding because people pressure them to "move on, put this experience behind, and go on." Without processing the feelings and thoughts of loss and grief, they cannot move through the healing process. Keeping the feelings inside and pushing away the thoughts may result in relational, physical, emotional, cognitive, and spiritual problems in the present, and lead to later difficulties in life.

This book is dedicated to the thousands of children, teens, and adults who courageously shared their pain, and their stories. They, the grievers, have been our best teachers at The Dougy Center.

Six Basic Principles about Children and Grief

1 *Grief is a natural reaction to loss.*

Grief is a natural reaction to loss. When a person dies, those who are impacted by the death experience grief. This is true for infants through adults, although the grief will vary from person to person. Grief does not feel natural, in part because we cannot always control our response or the experience. The sense of being out of control may be overwhelming or frightening, yet grieving is natural, normal and healthy.

2 *Each person's experience is unique.*

While many theories and models of the grieving process may provide a helpful framework for understanding grief, the path itself is a lonely, solitary and unique one for every individual. No book, article, or grief therapist can predict or prescribe exactly what a child, teen, or an adult will — or should — go through or experience. Those who wish to assist people in grief do best by walking with them, in the role of listener and learner, allowing the griever to teach them about his or her unique grief journey.

3 *There are no "right" and "wrong" ways to grieve.*

Coping with a death does not follow a defined pattern or set of rules. There is no "right" or "wrong" way to grieve. There are, however, "helpful" and "unhelpful" choices and behaviors. Some choices and behaviors are constructive, life-affirming actions, while others are destructive and harmful, causing long-term complications. Because the sheer pain of loss often feels "crazy," it may be challenging to decide which thoughts, feelings and actions are helpful, and which are not. Usually grieving children get plenty of advice from others about what they should and shouldn't do, feel, think and believe following a death. What they usually need more than advice is a non-judgmental, listening ear, helping them to sort through the options and alternatives.

4 Every death is different, and will be experienced in differing ways.

Children commonly react in different ways to the death of a parent, sibling, other relative, or friend. It makes sense — each relationship meets different needs and is uniquely personal. Some of the grief literature talks about loss in an almost competitive way as if some losses are worse than others. You may read that the death of a child is "the worst loss." Or that suicide is the hardest to "get over." Comparisons about which death is the worst are not helpful, and may lead to unrealistic expectations or demands. While an individual may speak for himself or herself about what he or she experiences, one cannot categorically say that any loss is worse than, or easier than, another.

Within a family each person may grieve very differently too. For example, one member may want to talk, another one may cry all the time, and another one may want to be alone. This can create additional stress and difficulty within an already-stressed family. Each person's way should be honored as his or her way of coping.

5 The grieving process is influenced by a multitude of issues.

There are many issues impacting how one reacts to a death. Some of these include: the strength of the social support systems available (family, friends, community, colleagues); the nature of the death and how the griever interprets that; whether or not there was "unfinished business" between the griever and the person who has died, and the previous nature of that relationship; and the emotional and developmental age of the griever.

6 Grief never ends. It is something you never get "over."

This is perhaps one of the least understood aspects of grief in our society. It seems most people are anxious for

> "I've had people say you've got to go on, you've got to get over this. I just want to shout 'you're wrong! Grief never ends.' I don't care what they say."
>
> — Philip, 13

us to put the loss behind us, to go on, to get over it. When a significant person dies, his or her death leaves a vacuum in the lives of those left behind. Life is never the same again. This doesn't mean life can never again be joyful, or that the experience of loss cannot be transformed into something positive. But grief does not have a magical ending time. People report pangs of loss, pain, or grief 40, 50 or 60 years after a death.

Stages Phases and Tasks of Grief

Over the years many professionals in the field of death and dying have attempted to formulate a model for reactions to dying and death. One of the first and best known is Elisabeth Kubler-Ross' model of five stages dying people experience: shock, denial, anger, bargaining, and acceptance. Kubler-Ross' pioneering efforts studying the experience of how terminally ill people grieve their impending death has often been misunderstood and misused by applying it to all grievers.

First, not all grievers experience each or all of the stages. For example, some people do not experience anger when someone dies. They are often told by well-meaning others that until they "get angry," they will never be able to move to the next stage and past the loss. This places an unfair burden on the vulnerable griever, and ignores one of the most basic principles of grief: **every person grieves differently.**

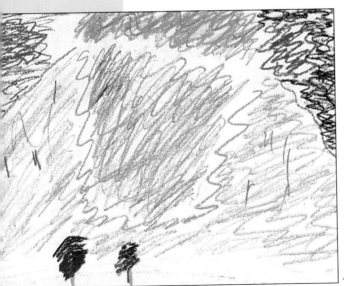

Second, many people have misinterpreted the stages as necessary and sequential — that one goes through denial, passing to anger, then bargaining, and so on. Kubler-Ross never intended the stages to be interpreted this way. Rather, she recognized that these stages were common to many terminally ill patients, and sometimes followed a pattern. But she did not imply there was a "right" or "wrong" way to grieve or that one stage would follow another.

Professionals in the field of death and dying have attempted to develop clearer and better models for understanding the grief process. Theories of "stages" and "tasks" of grief have evolved. Stage models concentrate on some of the common experiences of grievers and stages they may go through. Task models refer to what tasks the griever needs to accomplish to proceed in their grief work along the healing path.

As helpful as all of these models are, they often confuse rather than assist the grieving person, especially when attached to time frames. At The Dougy Center we have received dozens of frantic calls from grieving people over the years, terrified that their child or teen might have "missed a stage" and will have to go back and repeat it. Or they were told the stages take a year and then they'd feel better, but it's been a year and they don't feel better. Did they miss a stage or do it wrong?

Models of grief are often mistaken for a map of grief. They do not outline the route; each person must travel their own way alone. There are common experiences, and often grievers find that sharing their experiences with others is helpful. But remember: grief by its nature is individual, and follows an often unpredictable course.

Children tend to go in and out of grief.

The child's experience of grief often differs from the adult's in a significant way. While many adults describ the experience of grief as being in a fog for a period time, children seem to bounce in and out of the fee' of grief. Most children cannot sustain prolonged, periods of grief. They may be laughing one mir crying the next. This may be confusing to par other adults, as it is to the children themselv

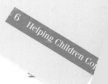

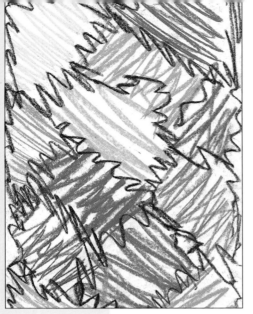

Not all children talk about their grief.

While adults and teens often talk about their feelings, thoughts and experiences following a death, not all children are able to—or choose to—process their grief verbally. Some are too young or developmentally immature to connect words with their feelings and thoughts. Others simply are not "verbal" children. Many children "act out" their feelings and thoughts through play and other actions. Some become withdrawn, angry, aggressive, tense, stubborn, defiant, or tearful. Children's primary mode of communication is behavior. Because grief is a powerful experience, it creates energy in the body. That energy needs a place to go or a way to be expressed. Children express that energy through play, in "high energy" activities like running and punching, and "low energy" activities like drawing or playing a game.

Some children don't seem to be affected at all.

Some children don't react much at all when they are told about a death. They may carry on with "life as usual," and show no outward signs of being impacted. Their actions or reactions do not necessarily give us an accurate picture of their internal experience. Some children are not able to pinpoint how they feel. Rather, they express that they feel "everything"—angry, sad, happy, fearful and hopeful, and occasionally that they feel "nothing"—listless, blah or numb.

Play is one way children make sense of their world.

Though some children may not verbalize, their feelings and thoughts frequently come out through play. Children attempt to make sense of their world through play; it is their work. When they paint or draw, put on puppet shows, dress up, or play in the sand, they are working out their internal experience.

Some children express their frustration and anger through hitting, biting or pushing, or hurting others. Some attempt to recreate a happier ending through playing the doctor who rescues the patient. Others take out their pain through hurting themselves, either for punishment or attention.

Four-year-old Jamie started attending The Dougy Center two months after his mother died of a heart attack. Over the thirteen months he participated, he would chose to go to the playroom and play with a wooden train set. He patiently connected the tracks in various configurations, thoughtfully assembled the train, and moved it around the tracks. Usually when it was time to go, Jamie would resist leaving. In the few sessions Jamie did not go to the playroom, he insisted on going upstairs and would run to the playroom and touch the storage box where the train equipment was stored.

One day the children were invited to bring memorabilia of the person who died, to share in a group with the parents. When it was Jamie's turn he shook his head, saying "I have a memory, but I'm not going to talk." We assured him he did not have to talk or share. As another child and mother shared a memory, Jamie whispered something in his father's ear. His father told the group that Jamie wanted him to share his memory. "Jamie remembers walking with his mom to the babysitter's house." Jamie interrupted him eagerly, continuing the memory. "Yep," he said. "There was train tracks there. My mom helped me walk on the tracks. Sometimes we waited for a train to come by, and we counted the cars." Then he smiled and sat down.

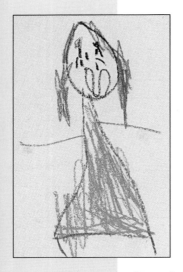

It's not unusual for children to experience physical reactions.

The pain of loss is physical as well as emotional. Many children and teens experience physical reactions following a death. These may include exhaustion/inability to wake up, or the opposite, restlessness and inability to sleep; stomachaches; headaches; nightmares; uncontrollable shaking; inability to concentrate or focus; regressive behaviors (bed wetting, thumb sucking, clinginess). Some may identify so intensely with the symptoms of the person who died that they begin to manifest similar symptoms.

Each of these is a normal response to a difficult situation. It's the body's way of saying, "Hey, I don't like this. I'm not going to go on with business as usual." While these reactions are normal, they may become problematic if persistent, severe and ongoing. If or when they interfere with healthy functioning for a prolonged period, professional intervention is recommended.

It's not unusual for children to experience difficulties thinking or concentrating.

Many children have difficulties with their thinking processes following a significant death. Some are unable to concentrate at school because their mental energies are focused on the loss and the changes that have occurred following the death. Many children have difficulties being attentive in a classroom situation. Their bodies are present but their minds are drifting to events and experiences not related to the classroom discussion, lecture, or project. Many children and teens have trouble completing homework because home is not what it used to be. Grieving children are doing grief work which requires a great deal of attention and energy. Some children and teens experience a decrease in their academic proficiencies and their grades go down. Some children work compulsively to gain approval or achieve perfection. Teachers will often say that the child is just using the death as an excuse not to do their homework, or to get attention.

The child or teen's developmental age will influence his or her reactions to the death.

Children have different capabilities for understanding and dealing with a loss, depending on their developmental and emotional age.

Their developmental age may be different from their actual age; we've all seen 12-year-olds going on 8 and 10-year-olds going on 16. But in general, children increasingly develop the capacity for understanding what death means, how it impacts them, and how to cope with it as they age. As they enter different developmental stages, they will need to renegotiate what the loss means to them now. For the 5-year-old whose mother dies, it means one thing at 5, another at 13, and quite another at 18. She will have to re-experience and reinterpret the death as she encounters new experiences without her mother, and as her emotional needs mature and change over time.

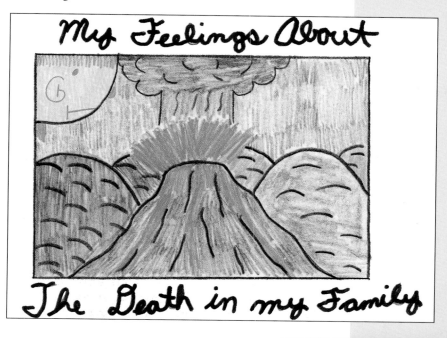

Behaviors may look different for different children and teens. Some become withdrawn and want to grieve alone; others become aggressive and act out their anger, frustration or other feelings. Still others become "very good." They may take on a parental role, trying to fill the void for their surviving parent and siblings.

It is not unusual or uncommon for children to believe they have seen or heard the deceased person.

Many children and teens talk about seeing the person who has died, or thinking they have seen the person or heard their voice. They may also have very vivid dreams where they interact with the person who is dead. This may be helpful to the child, or it may be frightening. Listening to their experience is important. It helps them to know these experiences are common and normal.

Understanding the Grieving Infant and Pre-schooler

Many adults underestimate the abilities of young children to realize something is wrong, and to understand what death is. As Alan Wolfelt, Ph.D., Director of the Center for Loss and Life Transition in Ft.Collins, Colorado states, "Any child old enough to love is old enough to grieve." A grieving infant may experience regressive behaviors

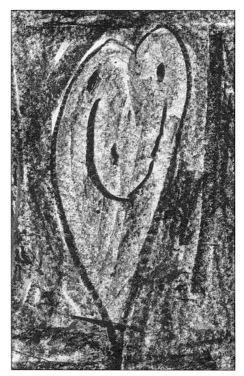

including changes in sleeping and eating patterns, clinging, or irritability.

Preschoolers often understand more than adults realize. Time after time a surviving parent has brought a preschooler to The Dougy Center, telling the staff member that the child didn't really know what had happened. Time after time, the child, upstairs in a play room, has told the story: "My mom got shot by a bad man and they can't find him. She's never coming back," or, "My daddy's heart got sick and broke and then he died. I miss him." Children are intuitive. They feel the trust in the atmosphere. They know something big has happened because the adults are acting different.

> *Provide the infant with as much routine and consistency as possible. He or she will also need lots of holding and comforting.*

Adults often talk around young children, believing they can't understand what is being said, or that they're too young to "get it." A grandmother whose husband was dying talked with her 32-year-old son in the car as her 3-year-old grandchild sat in the back seat. They spelled some words so the child wouldn't "catch on." When they arrived to visit grampa, the child ran into the house, jumped on grampa's lap and said, "Grampa — are you gonna be here for my birfday, or are you gonna be D-E-D?" Preschoolers have taught us they want and need to be told the truth, to be informed, and to have their questions answered truthfully.

It is important to understand that young children need to be included in the process when a family member is dying or has died. Attempting to "protect" them from this information will backfire in the long run, as they sense something is wrong yet no one will share with them what it is.

Children need clear, honest explanations about death

Although young children do not usually understand the finality of death, they can learn, over time, what it means. A 3-year-old, hours after being told her father is dead, asks her mother, "Is Daddy going to be dead all day?" When told

> *It is often helpful to have a pet funeral in which the child plans a "service" for the dead pet and actually buries it in a special place in the yard.*

his mother has gone to heaven, a 4-year-old wonders aloud, "When will she be back?"

Explaining death to young children is most helpful when it's simple and concrete. Explaining the finality of death to young children may include the basic, bodily functions: "when your mom is dead she can't eat, see, hear, sing, walk around, poop, laugh or cry. A dead person doesn't sleep, get hungry or cold or scared."

It may help if the child has a prior experience with death, like the death of a pet, or finding a dead bird on the lawn. Rather than hastily replacing the pet, or scooping up and tossing the bird, the parent can use these experiences as instructive and preparatory for children to understand death. Flushing a dead fish down the toilet may make a young child fear the "potty," or believe that's what happens to anyone who dies. Rushing out to replace a deceased dog may encourage the sense that the loved one can be easily replaced, and suggests that its uniqueness did not matter. Allowing a young child to experience the death of pets or other animals invites the curiosity of the child to be met with helpful explanations and information that can be applied when a more significant death occurs.

Ryan, 5, and Jeremy 4, whose fathers had died of cancer and suicide respectively, were playing in the backyard at The Dougy Center. Ryan hurt his finger and told the adult volunteer, "Look I've got an owie on my finger. I need a Band-Aid." While the adult was applying the Band-Aid, Jeremy whined, "I need a Band-Aid, too. I have an invisible owie." As a Band-Aid was being placed on his friend's invisible owie, the wisdom of childhood flowed from Ryan's mouth: "You know, at The Dougy Center everybody has an invisible owie because someone died."

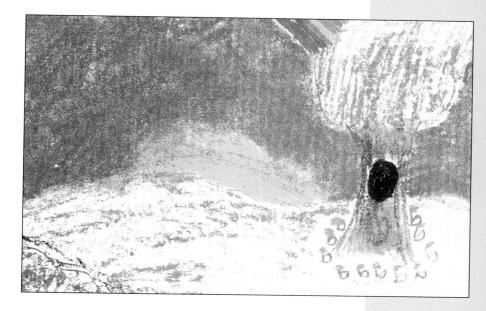

Young children may be repetitive in their questions.

It is common for little children to ask questions repetitively about the death. They learn about their world by having questions answered again and again. The same way that they learn 1 + 1 = 2, they learn about death through asking and getting answers.

Young children learn by repetition and therefore need to ask the same questions over and over, or to hear the story of what happened again and again, much as they like to be read a familiar bedtime story. This can be difficult, if not exasperating, for the parent grieving the death of a spouse or child.

A young mother called The Dougy Center concerned about her 4- year-old's morning ritual of wanting to watch home videos of the older brother who had died. She was concerned that this repetitive video watching would be

> *Reassure the children that there will always be someone to take care of them. Giving a child something that is important to you to hold until you get back may help the child feel more comfortable about your absence.*

harmful for her son. Also, it was difficult for her to see or to hear the video each morning. Following the video the boy would ask similar questions, but after hearing the mother's answers he would go about his play like any normal 4- year-old. Months later the child gradually discontinued his morning video watching and asking the same questions.

Young children don't necessarily have the tools to translate what they're feeling and thinking into language, although some are remarkably verbal and clear about what has happened.

After a death, a common fear of children is that others will die.

Because the death of someone close to a child upsets the sense of safety, security and control most children have, it is common for them to experience fear, insecurity and uncertainty.

> *"I don't want my mommy to ever be with anyone but my daddy. Daddy might be mad at mommy."*
>
> —Brittany, 5

Some children become very possessive of a surviving parent, afraid to let him or her out of their sight, terrified that he or she too will die or disappear. Some take the opposite behavior, seeming to not care about the parent, withdrawing from relationships with adults or other children. They may be fearful that anyone they get close to will die.

Some children are eager to help the surviving parent find a replacement for the deceased parent. A 5-year-old standing in the grocery line with his mother remarked to the male teller, "My dad died. Will you marry my mom?" Other children resent the time their surviving parent spends alone or without them; some children will do all they can to sabotage a potential relationship their parent might try to develop.

Most children in the 6-12 age range are still dependent on others for their survival and basic needs. The loss of a parent or sibling is confusing and difficult. Many children in this age group do not have ways to verbalize their complex and confused feelings and thoughts, which often come out as anger, frustration and irritability. Some children are very verbal and open to talking about how they feel and what they think, while others barely mumble in response to a direct question.

They tend to have magical thinking and often believe that they somehow caused the death. They frequently show signs of guilt because they assume that their behavior, thoughts or wishes contributed to the death.

Children in this age group want very much to be like their friends, and to fit in. They do not want to be different, yet when a parent or sibling dies, they **are** different. Often their friends, teachers, coaches and friends' parents don't know what to say or how to be around them.

Children in this age range respond well when they feel acceptance of their emotions and thoughts. Angry, frustrated children often do not know how to express those emotions except in behaviors that get them into trouble. It is helpful to assist them in finding ways to express this energy without hurting themselves or others. Suggestions include kicking nerf balls or a "kick box" rather than kicking another child or the dog. Hitting and pushing can be expressed with a punching bag or a stuffed animal. Children who need to bite can bite a rolled up hand towel. A "rage rag" (a rolled up hand towel with tape at one end and in the middle) becomes an excellent way to express anger by hitting something that represents how the person died such as a beer bottle, or the word "cancer" or "heart attack" written on a piece of paper.

Under-standing the Grieving 6-12 year old

> *"One day I got really mad at my mom cause she sent me to my room for a time out. I wished she were dead...and then she died."*
>
> —*Katie, 9*

Children are often tired and irritable because of sleeplessness, nightmares, night terrors, or staying up late watching television in an attempt not to be alone in their own bedroom. Many children want to sleep with or, at least, close to, the surviving parent. Some parents have found this comforting to themselves but become concerned about fostering unhealthy dependencies. Some parents find having a child sleeping with them is too disruptive of their own sleep so they arrange a place next to their bed for the child if she or he needs to come in during the night. Some parents prefer to stay in the child's room until he or she falls asleep.

It is important to help the child feel safe in whatever way the child prefers. Their fears won't last forever, and providing safety and comfort for the child in the ways he or she needs is critical.

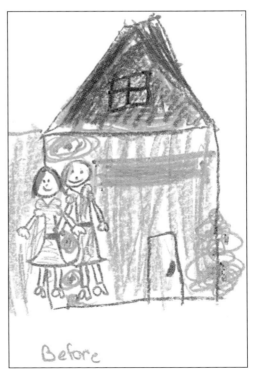

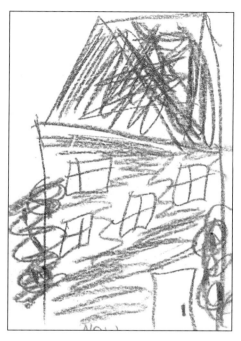

NOW

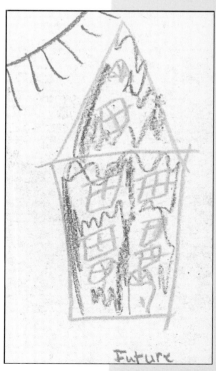

Future

Under-standing the Grieving Teen

Adolescence can be a difficult time even under the best of circumstances for most teenagers and their parents.

Adolescence is often a trying time for parents and their teenagers. The teenager struggles to find meaning, questions authority, tries to be independent while still reliant on others, weighs peer pressure, and juggles issues of dating and sexuality. Other teens and their parents may experience the adolescent years with more harmony and only minor difficulties. But the death of a significant person radically changes the anticipated future, relationships, roles, and the family structure of a young person.

Teens commonly think of themselves as immune from injury or death. When the death of a parent, sibling or friend occurs, the world as they understood it has been thrown into chaos. Many teens have difficulty communicating their thoughts and feelings about death with adults, especially the surviving parent, as they are also seeking independence from the parent.

As teens attempt to search for answers to their questions and struggle with the loss that has occurred, they may engage in behaviors that adults find frustrating: not communicating, not eating, skipping school, not doing homework, attempting to escape through alcohol or other drugs, acting out sexually, or exhibiting reckless behaviors.

Parents of teens often ask how to tell whether their teen's behavior is a result of the grief, or just typical teen behavior. If the changes have occurred only after the death, it is clearer that the death plays a major role in their behavior changes. Although it may be impossible to measure what part of their behavior is related to the loss and what part to adolescent struggles, in the long run it may not matter. Either way, they are struggling to make sense of the world and their place in it. Perhaps the best way to be of support is to listen, to be available, and approachable. As difficult as it may be, it is best to avoid, as much as possible, telling them what to do or what not to do. Allow the grieving teen to do his or her grief work as he or she chooses within reasonable boundaries.

The nature of the death.

How a child perceives and processes the nature of a death will impact how he or she deals with grieving. While it is frequently reported that children have a more difficult time if the death was by suicide or homicide, this is not always the case. Some children and teens are able to cope well with the suicide of a parent or sibling, while some who have had a parent or sibling die from a disease or accident are not able to cope as well. Some people believe that a sudden death is harder to deal with than a long-term chronic illness; others, that a long-term chronic illness exhausts the family over a long period of time and therefore is more difficult.

It is important to remember that the death a person is experiencing is the worst for them, and that comparisons about what might be worse or better are not helpful.

Issues of guilt and blame may be evident in any type of death. One 8-year-old girl suggested that the reason her mother was killed in a car accident was because she had taken her mother's favorite scarf to school that morning. Her punishment was the loss of her mother.

The response of the parent or parents.

When a parent experiences the death of a child or spouse, his or her parenting resources are drained. It is extremely difficult to cope with your own grief and "be there" for your children as well. Children often try to protect their surviving parent from more pain by "being extra good" or keeping their feelings inside. It is hard for them to see mom or dad cry.

This doesn't mean the surviving parent should not express emotion. Sometimes parents try to protect their children by being stoic, or crying out of sight only. It is okay for adults to express emotions in front of children; otherwise, children will never have healthy models for dealing with intense feelings. The adult should not, however, reverse roles and require the child to "take care" of him or her. Outside support systems, whether friends and family or a more formal support group, can help to meet the grieving adult's needs and allow for safe expressions.

Influences on How Children Cope with Death

Previous experiences with death.

Children who have had some experience with death prior to this death have developed some beliefs about death based on their own reaction and the modeling of others. Children learn by experience. Words like "dying" and "dead" are very difficult concepts to a young child with no prior experience of death. A child who has had an animal die better understands "gone," and the reality that the one who has died is not coming back. Deaths of pets or birds found on the lawn can provide good teaching opportunities for what it means to die, to be buried, and to be missed and memorialized.

For some children having experienced a previous death better prepares them for what to expect. For others, however, another death creates a feeling that everyone around them will die and their view of the world as unsafe is reinforced. They may become more fearful, stressed or anxious.

Support systems within and outside of the immediate family.

One of the dynamics within the family that often occurs following the death of a family member is that each person in the family experiences the death in a different way, and expresses their grief in a different way. Individual adults and children have had a different relationship with the person who died, therefore individuals have different thoughts and emotions about that person. Sometimes families recognize the value of differences, and are supportive to each other. Sometimes they do not allow for differences and judge each other's responses. And sometimes they protect themselves and each other by withdrawing, acting happy, or not mentioning the person's name.

> *"I wish my dad would talk to me about my mom. He just won't talk. And he tells me to shut up when I say anything. He was mad at me when I talked to my grandma on the phone."*
>
> *—Peter, 11*

It is not uncommon for families who have experienced a death to lose the contact and support of other family members — aunts, uncles, grandparents and step-families. Sometimes blame or bad feelings about the circumstances of a death, or the treatment of the person prior to death, splits families apart. This adds to the losses the children are experiencing.

> *"Coming to The Dougy Center really helps because all the other kids have had someone in their family die too. They really understand what it's like."*
>
> —Brian, 9

Support systems may include friends, relatives, neighbors, and members of clubs, organizations, and religious communities.

While the support systems of family, friends and community can be helpful, even families with strong outside support systems report that sharing with others in peer support groups like The Dougy Center is helpful.

Consistency and routines help during difficult times.

When a death occurs, other changes occur as well. The financial situation of a family may change dramatically, often for the worse, but even sudden wealth can bring problems because of the drastic changes. After parental death children may have to move to another city or home, change schools and leave friends, and take on additional responsibilities. Change is a loss, and all loss causes grief reactions.

Multiple changes put a lot of pressure on children (and adults) to adjust. Many changes often bring a lack of consistency in rules or in routine and may contribute to prolonging or complicating the grief process.

Special issues of homicide and suicide.

Many younger children do not have a complete understanding of suicide or murder, and don't think of it as "better or worse" than any other

> *"The thing that has changed the most since my mom died is that we're never home until after 8 o'clock. We always eat out after dad picks my little brother and me up. Then he wants to take us some place. I'm tired of getting home so late."*
>
> —Steven, 8

death. They simply focus on wishing the person were still alive. Others may understand and be able to process in a healthy way that the person suicided or was murdered. Young children tend not to have developed the "social

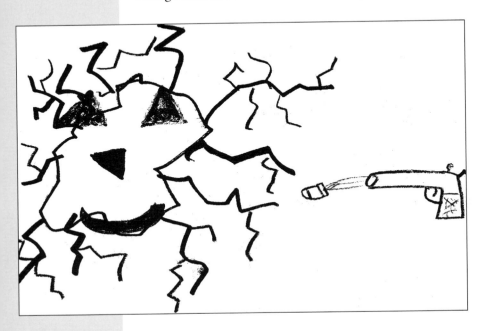

condemnation" or stigma of suicide or homicide. Unfortunately, our society tends to judge those who die by suicide or murder, and often by association, those who loved them.

Those who experience a death by homicide are often judged negatively by others. Sometimes people, in an effort to protect themselves from the possibility that a murder could happen to someone they love, believe that the murdered one's family must have in some way contributed to the event — that bad things happen to bad people. Obviously this attitude alienates those who are impacted by a homicide.

It is especially important to tell the children and teens how the person died, using words such as killed, murdered, suicided. Although using these words with children may be difficult, it is important for them to hear

I was happy, but then my life Got shattered

the truth from caring adults rather than from other children on the school grounds, or on the evening news.

Other factors that may make coping more difficult after a violent death are the impact of the media, and trial, if there is one. If the murderer is caught, there is someone to be angry at, but families seldom feel, whatever the verdict, that justice is done. Even if the accused is found guilty and sentenced to life in prison, he or she gets to eat, breathe and sleep, while the loved one is dead. If no one is ever caught, many children and teens express fear that the person will come and harm them.

Following a suicide, children may experience confusion about how and why someone could take his or her own life. It is important that they receive accurate information about what happened, and that their questions are answered honestly. Often they express a sense of feeling abandoned by the parent, sibling or friend who died by suicide. Because our society places a social stigma on the act of suicide, children may be teased or subjected to uncomfortable questioning. Being in a group with children who have had similar types of deaths helps to "normalize" their experiences. It is a practical way to reduce the effects of stigmatization and social isolation.

1 Sad.

2 Shocked.

.3. Angry.

4. louly.

Guilt

Many children and teens experience the complication of unresolved issues, guilt or unfinished business with the person who has died.

Young people are egocentric, and tend to believe the world revolves around them (which, in many cases, it does!). They may blame themselves for the death, or believe they somehow could have prevented it. Some have wished their parent was dead, and then when the parent actually dies, they believe they were responsible for the death.

While it is important to help children understand the death was not their fault, it may take time for them to express this concern, and to really believe they were not responsible. Their feelings should not be discounted. Asking children whether they think anything could have been done to prevent the death may uncover feelings of guilt. Responding in a way that discounts their feelings ("you shouldn't feel that way") may make them shut down rather than share what it's like to feel that way. Encourage them by asking clarifying questions around how they believe they were responsible, and gently help them understand the death was not their fault. It is helpful to talk to the child about the events surrounding the death and discuss what parts they could have controlled and which they really had no control over.

> *"I used to feel like it was my fault my father was killed. But talking with other kids helped me realize that it wasn't."*
>
> — *Mason, 14, whose father was murdered*

Anger

Many children and teens experience anger after the death of a parent, sibling or friend. The anger may be directed at specific others who "should" have prevented the death — a parent or doctor for example. Or it may be general anger that touches others randomly, sometimes for no apparent reason. It may be anger directed at God, at playmates, or at the surviving parent.

It makes sense that children and teens could be angry when someone they care about has died. It doesn't seem fair for a six- year-old to experience his father's death. Children see other intact families and remember fun times they had with their parent, and may feel angry at all the changes that the death has brought.

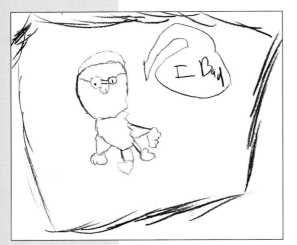

Most adults seem better able to deal with sadness in children than anger. They often have difficulty understanding that a child's anger is in part a reaction to the unfair situation they have been dealt in life. Children and teens need to be permitted to express anger in safe ways, and for it to be seen as healthy.

At The Dougy Center there is a room called the "volcano room," where children and teens can safely express the physical aspect of their emotions with the assistance of caring adults. The room's walls and ceiling are padded with 4" foam and covered with carpet. The floor has a 12" gym mat to cushion jumps and falls. Pillows, large stuffed animals and soft sponge balls may be thrown; a punching bag may be whacked. The "volcano room" concept can be adapted in many ways — kids can be encouraged to tear up telephone books, punch a pillow, get involved in sports, punch a punching bag, or a multitude of other physical activities that enable them to express their physical energy without hurting themselves or others.

Too often, children and teens are told they "shouldn't be angry." This only makes them angrier. Rather than try to take their anger away, we should attempt to find safe ways for them to express it verbally and physically. In the expression, it will dissipate.

Relief

Some children feel relieved after a death, especially if the person who died had been chronically ill or suicidal, requiring a great deal of attention and creating a tense atmosphere in the home. Children might feel relieved if the person who died was abusive, intensely angry, or creating a chaotic home environment. It is frequently difficult for children to talk about feeling relieved or glad when a person has died, as they may feel guilty. But it is important to allow for feelings of relief and gladness as well as sad or angry feelings.

Blame

After a death, children and teens often ask basic questions: why did this happen? Why did this happen to me? Sometimes blame can be placed on someone or something that contributed to the death — a drunken driver, an incompetent physician, an icy street.

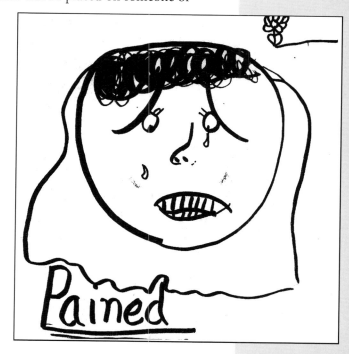

Sometimes blame is affixed on others who didn't have anything to do with the death. Some children blame the surviving parent. While this may not seem rational, the common saying "we always hurt the ones we love," may hold true. In their confused feelings, children and teens may be most unkind to those they know will continue to love them.

Denial

It is not unusual for children to experience denial about the death, whether at the time they are told, or even years later. Many people experience thinking "it is all a bad dream and I'll wake up and he'll be alive," or "maybe someday he'll knock on the door and be okay." This struggle is part of the normal process of coming to grips with the fact that the person will never be around again.

Persistent denial that the person is dead, or refusal to believe the death has occurred after a period of time may indicate that the child or teen needs help in his or her grief process.

Anxiety

Fear and anxiety are normal responses to a loss. The death of a parent or sibling upsets a child's sense of how things are "supposed to be." It forces them to think about the possibility that other people they care about may die, and that they may die. Their feelings of safety and security in the world are shattered. Sometimes this anxiety may come out through sleeplessness, fear of being alone, panic attacks, aggression, or inability to concentrate. These are normal responses, and, over time, with caring support, should diminish.

Some children are afraid to let their parent out of their sight and will move from room to room with them. They also may express reservations about going to school for fear that the surviving parent will die while they are gone.

Be honest.

Whatever you do, tell the child the truth. Do not lie about what happened. No matter how horrible the circumstances of the death are, children and teens need and deserve to know the truth. They should not be told someone died in a car accident if they died by suicide or were murdered. Many adults believe they are protecting children from the pain of the truth, when they are in fact protecting themselves. Denying a child the truth will ultimately cause the child more pain when the truth is discovered. Attempting to keep a "family secret" from the child will hinder open communication about grief issues.

> *"I'm really upset that my mom tried to hide the truth from me. I kept hearing her talk real quiet on the phone. I knew Jacob didn't just all of a sudden die. I thought maybe he died from a drug overdose. She lied to me as if I was some stupid kid."*
>
> —*Janette, 12*

It is not easy to tell a 10-year-old that her father shot himself, or an 8-year-old that his mother was murdered. But when children are not told the truth, they later resent not being respected enough to be told the truth. They tend to question whether or not they can trust any adult when the ones closest to them have lied to them. Most children will find out what happened even if they're not told by their family. Other kids will know, and eventually they will tell the grieving child, often in a hurtful manner. When they discover they have been lied to, they have another reason to be angry, and another complication to add to their already difficult lives.

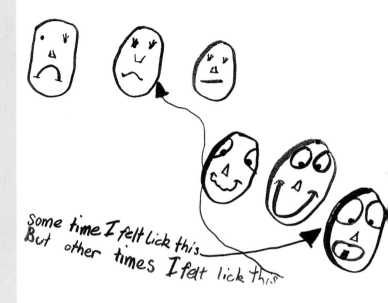

Some time I felt lick this. But other times I felt lick this

Use concrete language.

As much as possible, use the real words and explain what they mean when you discuss what has happened: dead, died, suicided, murdered. Although these words may seem harsh and stark, they assist the child in coming to terms with the reality of the death. When adults overuse terms like "expired," "passed," "passed on," "went to sleep," or the many other euphemisms so often used to cushion death's blow, children may be confused.

Answer the child's questions in language he or she can understand.

Parallels can be made between death education and sex education. A 4-year-old who asks, "How did daddy die?" and wonders, "How are babies born?" is not seeking a physician's report for the former or an exhaustive biological lecture on the latter. A good approach is to answer what is asked, naturally and honestly,

Jesse, six, was an avid reader. When he was told his grandfather expired in the hospital he replied, "Well, let's just go renew him."

without going into more detail than the child is seeking or capable of processing. Children are capable of understanding and processing more than many adults think. Children are curious and want to learn about death. Some children will ask more when they are ready, unless they learn that the subject is "taboo" or off limits.

Provide routines.

Routines allow grieving families to move through life in an acceptable manner while they are grieving. Routines also provide a safe, consistent environment for the children. They do not have to worry about what will happen to them and what each day will bring.

Allow choices.

When a death occurs children often feel and experience a lack of control. It helps in their healing process if they are allowed choices appropriate to their age and maturity level. Some children have difficulty making choices and are helped by being given options to choose from.

> "My grandparents are so stupid. They thought that I would believe my dad had died of a heart attack. My friend heard on the TV that my dad was shot by the police because he was drunk. He'd been in jail lots of times. I knew something bad would happen to him. Why did they lie to me? Even now they think I believe them."
>
> —Collin, 9

Allow children and teens the opportunity to be a part of the planning for funerals, memorial services, anniversaries and other decisions.

Too often children are excluded from the discussions or decisions regarding casket selection, burial versus cremation, memorial services and commemoration activities. The question is not should or shouldn't children participate in these decisions. The real issue is informed choice. They should be given a choice after the options are carefully explained to them.

Following the death of their father, 10-year-old Brian and 12-year-old Daniel were asked by their mother if they wanted to go with her to the funeral home to select a casket. Brian chose to go, and Daniel elected not to. Both boys are satisfied with their decision, and feel good about being given a choice. From our experience with thousands of children at The Dougy Center, the children without choice have more difficulty coping than those who received detailed information and were permitted to choose.

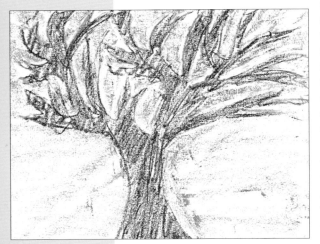

Eight-year-old Jacob went with his mother to pick out a casket for his 16-year-old sister who had died in a car accident. They narrowed the options to two, and Jacob took care to decide which casket he thought his sister would be "most comfortable in." He knew that his sister was dead, and therefore couldn't be comfortable or uncomfortable, but for him it meant something to be able to choose where he thought she would be most comfortable.

Children should be given choices as much as possible when a death occurs, for two reasons. First, having a say in what happens validates that they are impacted as much as the adults, that they matter, and that what they think and feel is important. Second, the ability to choose and influence decisions helps children regain part of the sense of loss of control which they often experience following a death.

Many people wonder whether it is harder for kids when someone is cremated than buried. Of the thousands of children who have participated at The Dougy Center, most have not had strong feelings about burial versus cremation, particularly if they have a place to go to remember the person who died.

Given an informed choice most children will want to see and to handle the cremains. The reasons for cremation and what the process is should be explained to children so they understand why and how the body is reduced to "ashes." Since children are concrete thinkers, seeing and handling the cremains helps them to deal with the finality of the death.

Five-year-old Brigitta announced to her friends at The Dougy Center that "Mommy let me and my sisters see daddy's ashes. We got to touch him too." Wide-eyed she explained, "You know, my daddy's ashes look like brownie mix with marshmallows." Then she smiled and returned to drawing.

Allow and encourage memorialization.

Allow children to have and display pictures, clothing

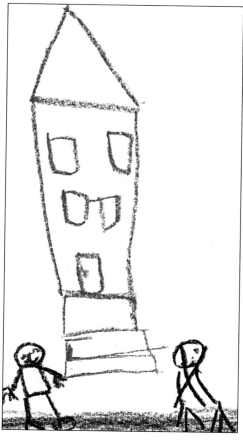

and other possessions of the person who has died. Some people believe it is best to get rid of everything that belonged to the person, and that hanging on to those mementos will only bring pain. Children should be given the choice to keep possessions and photos of the person who died.

Children are often not interested in the monetary value but the emotional, relational value of things. Smelly jogging shoes, a dirty apron, a worn Teddy Bear, dog-eared pictures, a used billfold are the everyday, used items that tend to be significant to children.

We suggest children and teens be included (if they choose to) in the process of sorting, keeping, and discarding the clothing and other possessions of the person who died. This allows the child or teen to continue to say "goodbye" in concrete ways. Also, the child or teen can select the things he or she most wishes to keep as memorabilia.

> *Five-year-old Brandi brought her father's black T-shirt to show her group at The Dougy Center. After she talked about her father and his favorite shirt, she held the shirt to her face and explained with a big smile, "It still smells like my daddy."*

Some children wish to have photos of the deceased displayed in the house, and others don't. Ten-year-old Joey and eight-year-old David experienced the death of both parents in a canoeing accident. Joey wanted the pictures of his parents left in the living room as they were. David didn't want any photos around because "it hurts too much." Their grandparents, who were their legal guardians, worked out a compromise with the boys, where some pictures were displayed in certain areas. The important part is to allow them to participate in these decisions.

Children often need opportunities for remembering the person who died. Putting together memory books is an activity that can be helpful in keeping the memory of the loved one alive. Children should be given the opportunity to do special things on holidays, birthdays and anniversaries, but should not be forced to participate.

Some children benefit from support groups where they can share with their peers.

Many children and teens can benefit from grief support groups with their peers. They often feel as if they are the only ones who have had someone die, and they feel isolated and alone. Sharing with peers may help to normalize their experience, let them know they're not alone or "crazy," and provide a safe environment to process their feelings. On the other hand, not all children or teens are prepared for, or responsive to, a group setting for dealing with their grief issues. At The Dougy Center we recommend that parents encourage their children to attend a group once, and if they choose not to return, their decision should be honored.

It is important to note that a child's ability to benefit from support groups is not dependent on wanting to talk about how they feel, or on playing well with others. At The Dougy Center we have had a number of children and teens who did not talk openly about their feelings or experience, and yet spoke before leaving about how helpful it was to listen and be able to make their own choices about sharing or not sharing. We have also had children who did not wish to be a part of our "opening circle," where each member of the group shares his or her name, who died, and anything about the death they care to share at that time. Even with an "I pass" rule allowing a child to pass without sharing, some children have chosen to sit outside of the circle, or in a corner. We allow and support their decision to be with the group and not part of it, and in most cases, eventually they join in and share their story in some way.

How do you know when a child or teen needs therapy or counseling?

When destructive or negative behavior is persistent or reoccurring, professional help should be sought. Most children and teens are "in and out" of their grief; that is, they experience sadness, anger and fear, but also are able to have fun and engage in activities. Prolonged or chronic depression, anger, withdrawal or fear may be indicators that the child needs some professional help in dealing with the loss.

If a child or teen is displaying severe reactions or disturbing changes in behavior, professional intervention is called for. Although it is not unusual for children or teens to talk about wanting to join the deceased, or to

How
to
Know
When
Professional
Help is
Needed

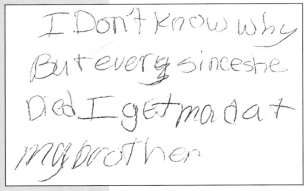

I Don't know why But every since she Died I get mad at my brother

die, any signs of self-destructive behavior or language about killing one's self should be taken seriously.

If a child or teen is experiencing physical pain or problems and doctors have not found an organic reason for the pain, professional help may unlock the key to the cause. Having physical symptoms following a death is not unusual; if they become problematic or debilitating, professional help should be sought.

Pitfalls to Avoid

Don't say you know how they feel.

Even if you have experienced a similar loss, you don't know how anyone else feels. Every person is unique and their experience of grieving is different from yours. You can say you also had your father die when you were a child, and you know something about what that's like. But don't say "I know how you feel." Rather, say, "tell me how you feel," or "I am here to listen if you want to talk about the death."

Don't tell them what to do unless they ask for your advice.

Many adults jump in too quickly to try to "solve" a child's problems, or tell them what they should or should not do. Most children, and nearly all teenagers, resent this. Help them come to their own decisions and conclusions by listening, and by helping them look

> *"I feel really angry when someone says, I know just how you feel — my great-grandpa died, or my dog died. They don't know what it feels like to have your mom murdered."*
>
> *—Marilyn, 15*

at the options available to them. On the other hand, if they ask for your advice, give it honestly.

Don't patronize them by saying trite things.

Don't tell a child he or she was lucky to have his mother or father for as long as he or she did. Don't tell them they'll be all right in a year or two. Don't try to take their pain away by saying things intended to "solve" or take away their pain.

Don't say "You're the man (or woman) of the house now."

Boys whose fathers die and girls whose mothers die continue to be told by well-meaning but uninformed adults that they are now the man (or woman) of the house and need to take good care of their mother (or father.) This puts children and teens in unrealistic roles, with impossible tasks. Children are children, and need to be able to be children. They should not have to parent a parent, or parent their siblings.

But I don't know what to say!

It is not what you say that matters to a grieving person as much as your openness to listening. Most people do not remember the things that people say to them in the days following a death (unless they are hurtful or insensitive — then they remember.) They remember who showed they cared, who listened, and who was available to be with them. Too many people try hard to make grieving children and adults "feel better," and it often backfires.

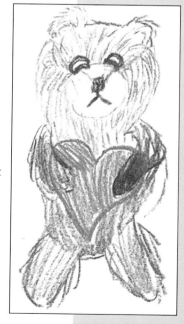

When you truly don't know what to say, say that! Say, "I don't know what to say. There are no words that can bring your father back, but I want you know that I care and want to help in any way I can."

Children and teens often say that people were there for them for a week or two after the death. In the days and months following the death it is helpful to call and/or send an "I'm thinking of you" note. It is a very lonely journey and the support of friends helps.

Dealing with the Spiritual Aspects of Death

Is it okay to tell children their loved one is in heaven?

If your religious belief system includes a heaven, yes, it is perfectly appropriate to tell a child his father is out of pain and is in heaven with God. Young children may still have difficulty understanding the concept of heaven (it may seem no different than the last business trip mom or dad went on). A way to explain it is this: " We believe that Dad went to heaven when he died. So his body doesn't work any more and is dead, but his soul is in heaven with God."

It is generally not helpful to children or adults to say things like "God wanted him." The child may think "so did I!" and be resentful of God.

What about God?

For those families whose spiritual beliefs include a belief in God, there are often complications in understanding how the God they have believed in could allow the death to happen. Many children and teens feel anger toward God for allowing their loved one to die. They should be allowed to explore their feelings without judgment, and be permitted to work through why God would allow the person to die when they feel like they needed him or her in their lives.

How do I tell my children about a death?

Children and teens have taught us at The Dougy Center that they want to be informed of deaths quickly, honestly and completely, face to face. They want their questions answered truthfully with the best information the adult has. If you don't have all of the information they ask, simply tell them you don't know, but that when you do you will let them know.

Don't lie, sugar coat the truth, tell half-truths or provide partial explanations. When adults withhold information about questions children are asking, they are teaching children that adults will not be truthful with them. It may be difficult to answer their questions completely and truthfully, because often the information they ask is painful and difficult for you as well. But your children will hear rumors, or the truth, from other children or adults, and it is important that they hear it honestly from you in order to be able to trust you and what you tell them.

It is best to have someone the children know share this news. We are sometimes asked by callers to The Dougy Center if a staff person could, for example, tell the children in a family that their father has died. Although there may be a rare occasion when this is appropriate, in general it is better for them to hear from people they know and trust. Sharing it with them with the support of a close family friend may be okay, but it should be someone the children feel comfortable with.

Should the children attend the funeral?

Children should be allowed the choice of whether or not to attend a funeral or memorial service, after you fully explain what will happen there in a way they can understand. For example, you can explain that a funeral is a way to celebrate the life of the person, and also a way to express our sadness over missing them. You should explain that people may be crying, and the person will be lying in a box called a casket. Let the child know that the person who died may look a little different than we remembered. Inform the child specifically about the casket, viewing the person, and other details of the service.

Common Questions about Children and Grief

Be aware that a child may change his or her mind within minutes of the service. Knowing this, it is important to have alternate plans arranged. A child may also change his or her mind in the middle of a service, so prior arrangements should be made for an adult to be with the child if he or she has questions or wants to leave. This designated person can provide a comforting presence so the parent or parents can be present at the service, and the child can leave without being reprimanded.

My child doesn't seem to be grieving, and I haven't seen her cry. How can I help?

First, it is important not to associate "grieving" with crying. Not all grief is displayed in sorrow and tears. Children often hide their feelings from adults, sometimes in an effort to protect a parent. Some children do not cry, but that doesn't mean they are not grieving. Adults

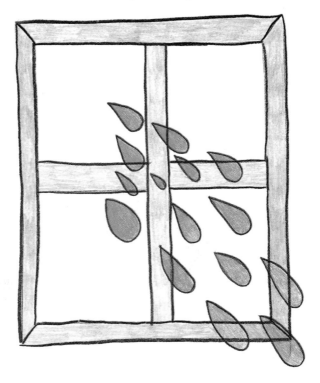

should provide an atmosphere where it's safe for children to share feelings or not share them. You can help your child by understanding that she is grieving, but is not expressing that with tears just now. You can help her by allowing her to grieve and express that grief in her own unique ways. And you can help her by removing your own expectation that she should or needs to cry.

Adults can set a good example for children by being free to express emotions without putting children in the position of needing to take care of them. Letting a child know it's okay to cry and showing that by example may provide the "permission" a child needs to share feelings openly.

How do I get my child to talk about the person who died?

Most children work through their grief through their play. It is best not to try to force your child to talk about the person who died, but to allow for those opportunities and to set a good example. You should talk about the person who died, using his or her name, sharing memories. It is helpful to spontaneously mention things about the person who died when you think of them. For example, if you're passing a favorite restaurant, instead of tightening up and looking the other way, you might say, "Hey, kids, your dad and I loved the Caesar salad at that place." This allows them the freedom to bring up other foods, other memories, and other issues about the person who died. If and when the child is comfortable, he or she will talk about the person as well. Sometimes it will take time for them to be able to do so. If you push, pressure, manipulate, or try to force your child to talk, you will probably push him or her further away.

It may be that you have a need to talk about the person who died, but your child doesn't at this time. Children often want to hear others reminisce, but do not choose to do so themselves. Some children are confused because a surviving parent is pressuring them to talk, but is unwilling to talk about their own thoughts and emotions. Others may be resentful because when they did talk, they were criticized about what they said with comments like, "That's not true," or "You shouldn't feel that way." Some children protect their private thoughts because they are convinced adults will not accept them or will try to change them.

My child's grades are slipping — how can I get him to focus on his schoolwork?

During the initial stages of grief many children have a great deal of difficulty listening, sitting still, and concentrating. This is normal in the grief process. You may want to talk with your child's teacher and see if he or she will ease up on the required work, or allow for choices that make it more relevant to your child. For

> "My grades started getting better after my teacher asked me if I wanted to bring a picture of my dad to school. I left the picture in my desk, and felt like my dad was helping me through the day."
>
> —Jeffrey, 9

example, writing a biography of the person who died may be of great interest, but writing about George Washington is of no interest. A health assignment may focus on the disease of the person who died rather than some obscure health issue unrelated to the child's experience. Finding a buddy in class who can help the child stay current on assignments and get help when needed may be beneficial.

We think teachers and principals need to be aware of the long-term effects of grief, and to be creative within the classroom and school in providing opportunities for its expression. Children will thrive in a supportive, creative educational environment that acknowledges the death and gives them options around processing their grief.

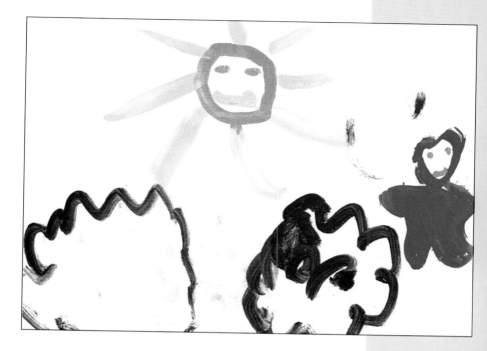

My child has nightmares and sleeping problems since the death. Should I let her sleep with me?

Your child may be fearful that something bad will happen to you during the night, or that you will die too. Nighttime is a time when the distractions of the day are gone and thoughts about the person who died may flood in. These thoughts can make it difficult to get to sleep, or to stay asleep.

It is okay to comfort her in whatever ways you feel comfortable. You may choose to stay with her until she falls asleep in her own bed, or you may allow her to sleep with you or in a bed beside you. You may also consider giving her something special to sleep with, like a Teddy Bear. Usually these fears will subside over time and she will want to return to her own room.

"I like sleeping in my mommy's old sheets. I feel close to her and I don't have nightmares anymore."

—Kim, 7

My child seems overprotective of me and won't let me of his sight. What can I do?

It is not uncommon for children to be worried about others dying when a parent or sibling has died. It is important for your son to know where you are, what your plans are, and when you intend to return. If any changes in that plan occur, you should let him know, even if they seem minor to you. Even if a parent is 10 minutes later than planned, children can become very fearful and fantasize about what could have happened to you. Check in with him frequently, and provide him with hugs, and assurances that you will stay in touch with him. Let the child know he can call you if he needs to check in. Be careful not to say that nothing will happen to you, because you can't ensure that nothing bad will occur.

My child doesn't seem to be eating well. What can I do?

Many children experience eating difficulties during their grief process. Some seem to lose all interest in food, while others overeat. If your child is not eating, offer small amounts of food frequently during the day rather than three larger meals. Letting your child plan or have input into what foods he or she would like could help in regaining an appetite. It is especially important to drink healthy fluids (milk, water, juices) during this time.

If your child is overeating, or eating only junk foods, make sure you have healthy quick snacks, like fruit, available. [Hint: cut or slice the fruit up and it is more likely to be eaten.] Try to provide healthy meals. Many families do not maintain healthy cooking or eating habits following a death because it seems to take too much energy. Families at The Dougy Center frequently report that many of their meals are from fast food take-outs, which are often high in fat and low in nutrition. Although it may be difficult for you to prepare or ensure nutritious meals, especially if you have your own eating difficulties, make an effort to do so for your child's health and welfare.

Should I let my child see the deceased's body at the funeral home?

Children at The Dougy Center have taught us that they want to make that choice for themselves. A child can make the choice that is best for him or her after being informed about the condition of the body, the location of the body, and what they might see. We suggest children be allowed to see the deceased when only one or two adults are in the viewing area. Many children ask questions or want to do things that are uncomfortable for some adults.

Be aware that your explanations may be confusing. Try to avoid jargon. Make your explanations as easy and simple to understand as possible. For example, most people refer to the viewing of a deceased person as "viewing the body." Children may interpret this to mean that there is no head, and be terrified to see it.

Amber, 5 and Amy, 4, were told in detail about their father and what it meant for him to be dead: that he "can't breath, move, or talk." They were told he would be in a casket ("like a big shoe box") at a funeral home ("big building"). They had already chosen to see

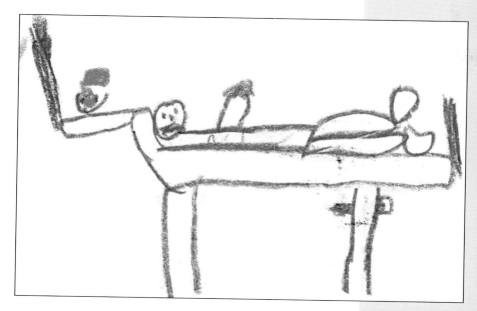

pictures of the wrecked family car in which their father had died. At the funeral home, they ran holding hands up to the casket standing on tiptoes to see their dad. "Why are his hands so cold?" Amber asked her aunt. "Does he have his shoes on?" asked Amy, peaking under the satin liner. After many questions and truthful answers, the girls climbed on chairs to kiss their father and said, "Goodbye, daddy." As they left the funeral home they talked about going to the ice cream parlor to buy their dad's favorite flavor.

Remember:

The most important thing you can do to help a grieving child is to provide a safe, supportive environment where you include the child in decisions, listen to his or her fears and feelings, and respect his or her experience by being truthful.

The mission of The Dougy Center is to provide loving support in a safe place where children, teens and their families who are grieving a death can share their experience as they move through their healing process. The Dougy Center extends supportive services to the family, caregivers, schools, businesses and the community.

The Dougy Center serves children and teens ages 3-19 who have experienced the death of a parent or sibling (or, in the teen groups, a friend), to accident, illness, suicide or murder. The support groups are coordinated by professional staff and trained volunteers. In addition, the parents (or caregivers) of the youth participate in support groups to address their needs and the issues of raising children following a traumatic loss.

When The Dougy Center was established in 1983, it was the first of its kind in the country. In response to numerous requests for information about our program, The Dougy Center developed a training and publications program to help other communities establish centers for grieving children and families. Through our National Center for Grieving Children, The Dougy Center has trained individuals and groups throughout the world, and now publishes a National Directory of Children's Grief Services, updated annually.

The Dougy Center is a 501(c)3 nonprofit organization and raises its entire budget from individuals, businesses and foundations. We receive no government funding, or third party payments. Participating families may contribute to the program, but there is no fee for service. While families receiving services contribute what they can, many do not have the financial resources to pay anything. Since The Center will never turn a family away because of their inability to contribute, we are totally reliant on private support from our friends in the community.

How can I support The Dougy Center or get additional information about your programs?

Contributions to The Dougy Center are tax-deductible to the full extent allowable under IRS guidelines. Your gift can be made out to The Dougy Center and mailed to us at the address below.

You can receive additional information about:

- Other Guidebooks available from The Dougy Center
- Videos and other resource materials available from The Dougy Center
- Obtaining the National Directory of Children's Grief Services
- Program development training at The Dougy Center's annual Institute in Portland
- How to schedule a training or presentation in your area
- Supporting The Dougy Center through a will or bequest

Write or call:

The Dougy Center
P.O. Box 86852
Portland, OR 97286

Phone: [503]775-5683
FAX: [503]777-3097
e-mail: help@dougy.org
Website: www.dougy.org

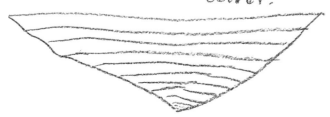

I like Duggy Senter very much.
I like shering my feelings
it makes me feel Better.

Development of this Guidebook was made possible through a grant from the **Meyer Memorial Trust.**

The Guidebook was printed through the generosity of **Western Lithograph.**

Contributors to the Guidebook include:

The Dougy Center staff —

Donna L. Schuurman, Ed.D.,
  Executive Director/Lead Writer

Joan Schweizer Hoff, M.A.,
  Associate Director/Writing & Editing

Donald W. Spencer, M.Div., M.Ed., M. Coun.Psy.,
  Director of Family Services/Writing & Editing

Cynthia White, M.A.,
  Training Director/Writing & Editing

Stephen Guntli,
  Director of Development & Planning/Editing

Kellie Campbell,
  Administrative Support/Editing

Design: **Fitzsimon GRAFIX / Fran Fitzsimon**

Cover Art: **Debra Hunt**

Inside Art: **Provided by children from The Dougy Center**

  The Dougy Center could not exist without the generous contributions of **hundreds of volunteers** who give of their time, boundless energy, unflagging enthusiasm, and matchless dedication. We thank them for accompanying the children, teens, and adults who come to The Dougy Center in their grief journey.

Additional Resources to Explore

Healing the Bereaved Child,
Alan D. Wolfelt, Ph. D., Companion Press, 1996.
(Available by calling 970/226-6050)

Life & Loss: A Guide to Helping Grieving Children,
Linda Goldman, Accelerated Development, 1994

Are You Sad Too?
Helping Children Deal with Loss and Death,
Dinah Seibert, M.S., Judy C. Drolet, Ph. D., and Joyce
V. Fetro, Ph. D., ETR Associates, 1993

Talking About Death:
A Dialogue Between Parent and Child,
Earl A. Grollman, Beacon Press, 1990

The Grieving Child,
Helen Fitzgerald, Fireside Publishers, 1992

Notes